Authors: Sandy Chubb   Sister Elaine MacInnes

Freeing the Spirit...

ries and Info

2015

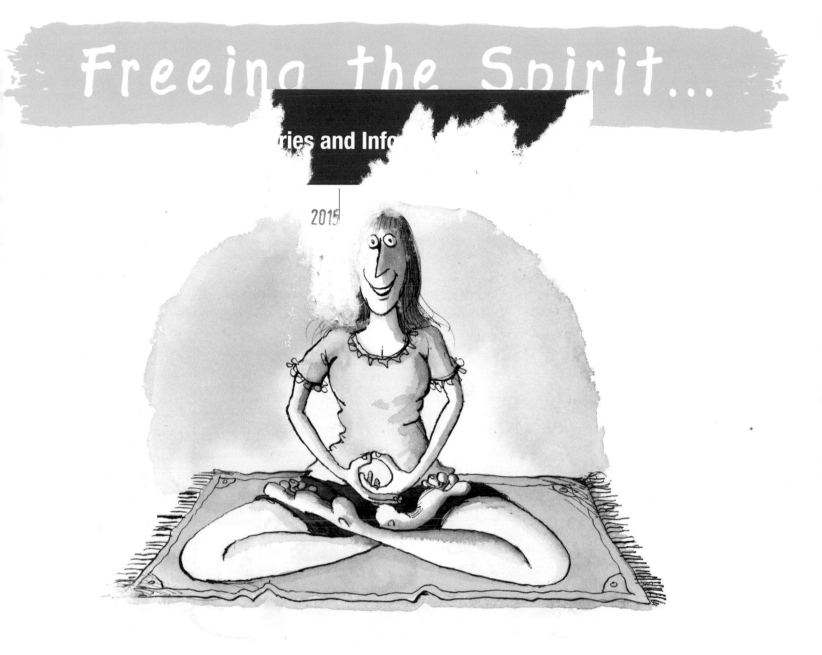

...through meditation and yoga.

Editor: Susanna Lee   Illustrations: Korky Paul

Design: Nicola Kenwood

BODY PARTS

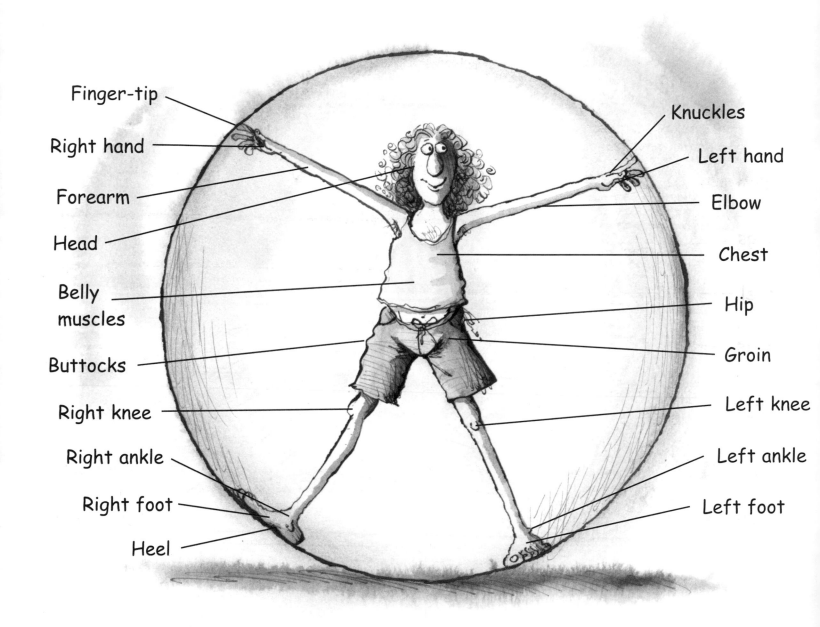

Finger-tip

Right hand

Forearm

Head

Belly muscles

Buttocks

Right knee

Right ankle

Right foot

Heel

Knuckles

Left hand

Elbow

Chest

Hip

Groin

Left knee

Left ankle

Left foot

BODY PARTS

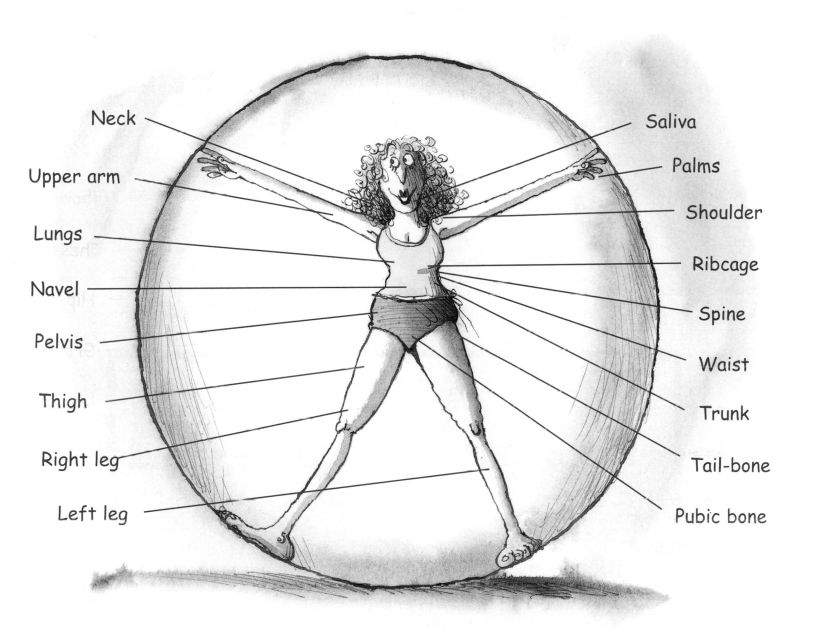

Neck

Upper arm

Lungs

Navel

Pelvis

Thigh

Right leg

Left leg

Saliva

Palms

Shoulder

Ribcage

Spine

Waist

Trunk

Tail-bone

Pubic bone

Important!

If you get stuck on any of the new words in this book,
look in the 'glossary' in the back for help.

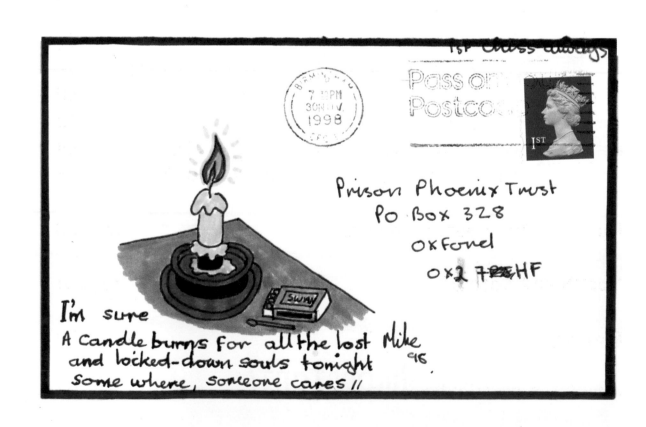

CONTENTS

Introduction   page 10

Part 1   **Let's start with yoga**   page 11

Healing stress in prisons   12
Poses – Asanas   13
Breathing practice – Pranayama   14
So what's the problem?   16
How to start   21

Part 2   **Let's move on to meditation**   page 23

Why meditate?   24
How to sit in meditation   26
How to silence the mind with breath counting   34
Difficulties you may find in meditating   40
The effects of meditation   42
Suggested prayers before and after sitting   44
How to make a zafu and meditation bench   46

Part 3   **Yoga poses – Asanas**   page 50

Health and Safety   page 51

Glossary   page 95

About the contributors   page 98

Dedicated to all members
of the prison community and
all imprisoned people
everywhere

An offering towards peace of mind.

To the memory of
Ann Wetherall

1924 - 1992

Founder of the Prison Phoenix Trust

and to the memory of
George Spence, former life prisoner
and long-term friend

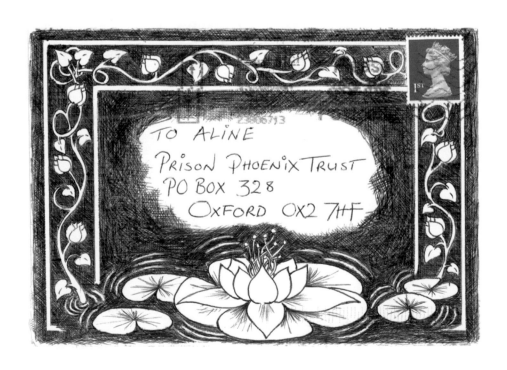

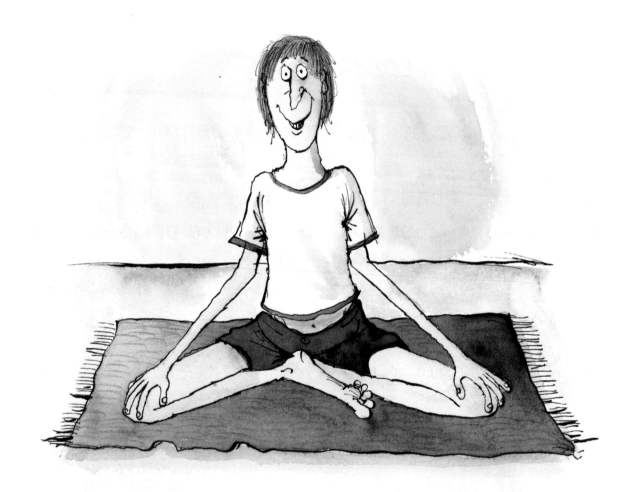

About this book

This book gives easy-to-follow guidelines on how to do meditation and yoga in your cell.

**Yoga and meditation help us all alike –
the captive and the free.**

About the Prison Phoenix Trust

The Prison Phoenix Trust has worked in prisons for 18 years. Every season we send out newsletters to prisoners who have been in touch with us. Each month we hold workshops in prisons all over the country. Every day we write to give support in meditation and yoga to people who are captive.

If you would like some help with your practice and would like to receive our Newsletter, please write to us!

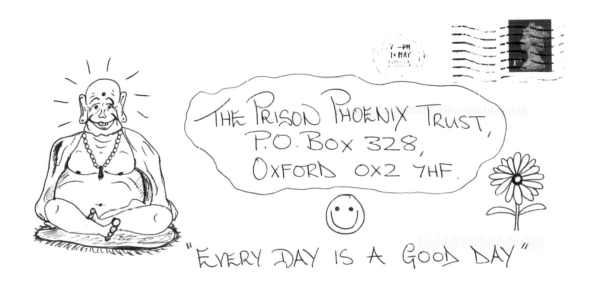

THE PRISON PHOENIX TRUST,
P.O. BOX 328,
OXFORD OX2 7HF.

"EVERY DAY IS A GOOD DAY"

Introduction

The Prison Phoenix Trust (PPT) helps prisoners to turn their lives around by using their cells as places of spiritual practice.

The PPT works with prisoners of any religion – or none at all – because everyone can grow through yoga and meditation.

The practice of yoga helps you become steady, calm, quiet and comfortable. Doing yoga improves your health and helps your body fight disease.

Meditation helps us discover who we really are. We learn to feel better about ourselves and the world we live in.

Yoga silences the body.
Meditation silences the mind.

Let's start with yoga

Yoga was in India as long as 5000 years ago. The word 'yoga' means experiencing oneness. With practice, we awaken to the fact that body and mind are one.

Then you can experience being connected with everything in Creation. This feels very refreshing.

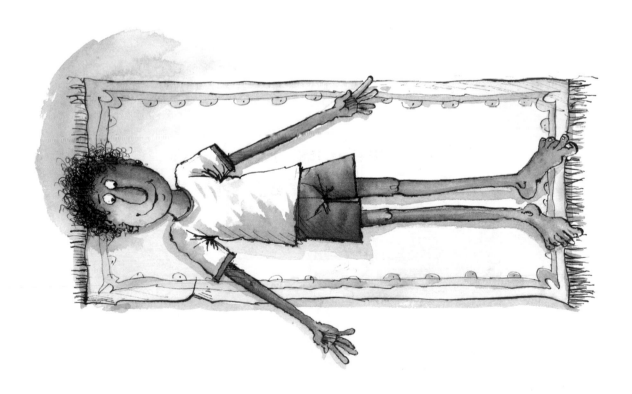

Healing stress in prisons

When we go to prisons we often hear "I'm stressed out and I can't get my head together".

How can any of us get our heads together when our bodies are full of physical tension - or when we sleep badly because our heads keep racing and the body gets more and more wound up?

Many of you in prison work out with weights or do gym. Sometimes this doesn't help enough. Weights and gym are great for getting fitter but they don't always relax or heal in the way that prisoners need.

Yoga can heal and relax you at a deeper level.

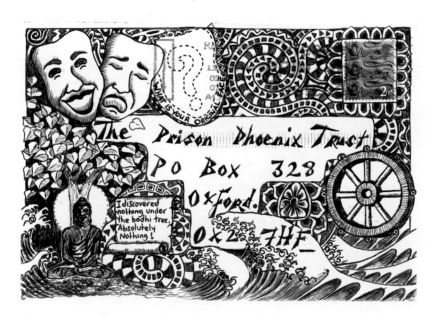

Poses - Asanas

Yoga exercises are called Asanas.

Each pose is held for a number of seconds. The practice of yoga begins when we learn to relax and be still in each pose.

Then we can concentrate on the breath. Everything starts to work properly, from the glands to the nervous system to yourself.

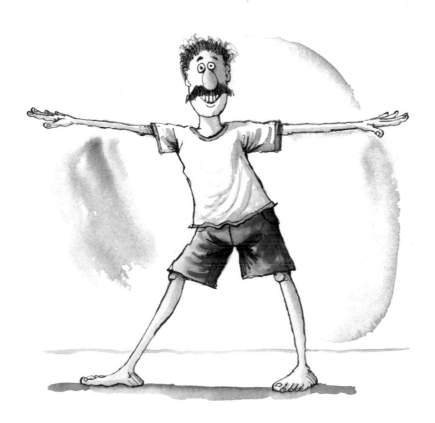

Breathing practice - Pranayama

Breathing practice in yoga is called Pranayama.

The breath is so important. For hundreds of years yoga teachers have taught that working with the breath can:

- help spiritual growth
- help clear our thinking
- help bring happiness
- help us act well towards others
- help calm the nervous system
- help purify cells in the body
- help ease depression

Try taking a few breaths the Yoga way

- breathe in and out through the nose if you can
- be aware of the air filling the bottom of your lungs, then the middle and then the highest part
- hold the breath for a second or two and then release easily
- when the lungs are empty, relax and pause
- when it happens naturally, breathe again

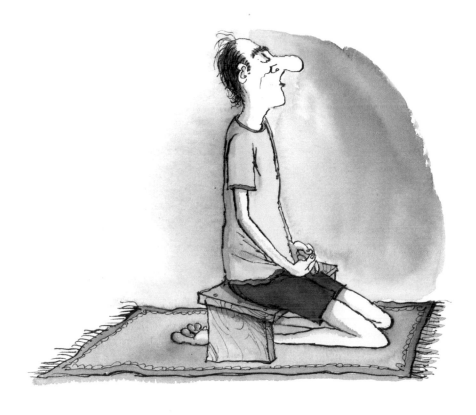

So what's the problem?

1. "I can't concentrate for two seconds, let alone twenty"

When you focus on the breath – its sound, its length, the space it fills - it is surprising how quickly time passes.

Asanas are the key to learning how to make the most of vital energy. Instead of wasting time and energy you learn to redirect it. You will find that you can sit still for long periods of calm.

2. "Yoga is for weirdos, women and wimps..."

Some men and women spend a lot of time down the block in tough prisons. They often say that all the energy they put into violence is a sort of self-protection.

When you learn to transform that energy you become more powerful.

You can lead a happier, healthier, calmer and more sociable life.

Far from being a wimp, you gain more self-respect and other people start to respect you more.

Find this out for yourself....

3. "I'm a dope user, heavy smoker and I'm unfit. I never stick at anything......."

You can change the negative picture you have of yourself.
One reason some people get sick is because they can never see themselves as well people. Picture yourself well and happy.

People do yoga because it makes them feel good.

You'll find that bad habits give you up, and however stiff you are, you'll get more supple.

Try it – just for a month.

4. "I'm in a small cell and there's no room"

Most yoga mats are two feet two inches by six feet (66cms x 1.83m). That's all the space you need to work on.

You don't need a mat by the way, just a floor you don't slip on.

Try the poses in bare feet. This is the yoga tradition.

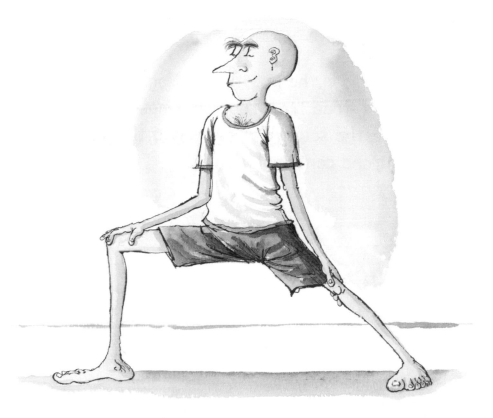

The words of some Hindu spiritual teachings

The Upanishads – say this:

"When the body is in silent steadiness, breathe rhythmically through the nostrils with a peaceful ebbing and flowing of breath. The chariot of the mind is drawn by wild horses, and those wild horses have to be tamed."

"Find a quiet retreat for the practice of Yoga, sheltered from the wind, level and clean, free from rubbish, smouldering fires and ugliness, and where the sound of waters and the beauty of the place help thought and contemplation".

How to start

Here are some things you can do to help:

- check your small floor area is clean

- if possible get some fresh air in - open a window - change the air in your lungs

- if you smoke, clean the ashtray

- bring nature to your cell - a leaf, twig or stone from outside – make your own Sacred space by placing a precious and personal object on a clean handkerchief or paper tissue

- look out of the window if you have one - tune in to the clouds and sky before you begin

- doing yoga in the morning when the mind is most clear is best – but work gently until your body loosens up.

- start your yoga in warm loose clothes – not jeans

In-exhale

Wise men travel many miles
Wise women sail the seas,
A wise man can fly many days
To find a well-wise tree,
Intellectuals and scholars
Find it so hard to believe,
It's not about location
It's about the way you breathe.

The body that wins prizes
Cannot sustain the dream,
The protein and the vitamins
Will never reign supreme,
Every mirror that is made
Is programmed to deceive,
It's not about the muscles
It's about the way you breathe.

Sometimes there is confusion
Between the left and right,
Sometimes you'll find we all look out
When we need insight,
But once you have found balance
It's easy to conceive,
It's not about resistance
It's about the way you breathe.

It's folly to take simple verse
And make them complicated,
The humble breath does not need
words
To be communicated,
When big ideas have come and gone
There is no need to grieve,
It's not about great speeches
It's about the way you breathe.

Benjamin Zephaniah ©

Benjamin Zephaniah, famous poet, PPT Patron and former prisoner,
wrote this poem for prisoners reading this book.

Let's move on to meditation

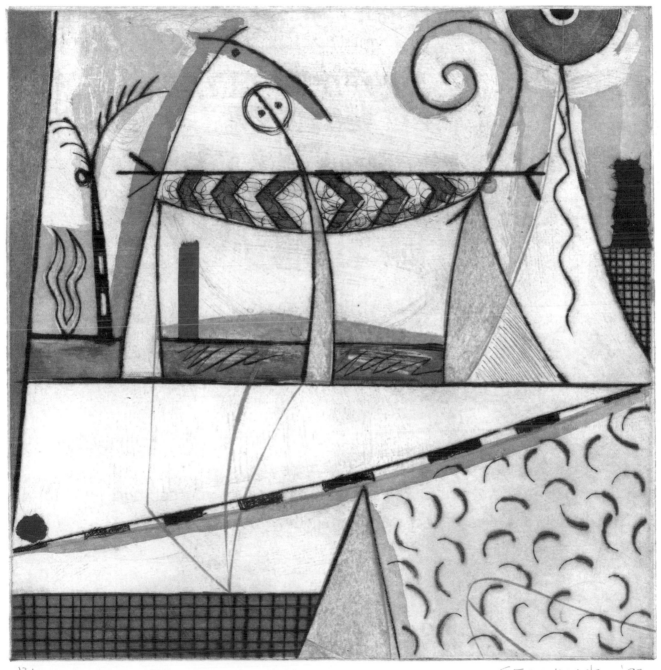

13/20   Susan Moxley '98

Why meditate?

Getting a sense of life and light

Monks and nuns, as well as prisoners, have homes called cells.
When a person chooses to go to a cell they want a time for silence
and reflection. They seek time to deal with pain and darkness.
They want time to get closer to understanding. They want to feel a
sense of life and light.

The sleeping child

Meditation can help you find who you are inside. Some people say
that finding the real self is like being put in touch with a small
sleeping child. When you find your child inside you can nurse him or
her through the ups and downs of living.

Our own healing breath

When we work with our breath we are working with the Life Force itself. This is both powerful and sacred.

Let the power in the breath do its own thing for you. It will shift the blocks that stop your head working the way it should.

Our meditation is very simple. First silence the body by moving into the right position. Then silence the mind through focus on the breath.

Sitting in silence brings automatic effects. Meditation is not easy. You can't blot out unhappiness. But you will find some things about yourself that you can love. You can also come to terms with your past.

For thousands of years meditators have known that we all have an inner power. If we allow it to heal body and mind by sitting in silence we can change our lives. But we have to do that for ourselves.

How to sit in meditation

Getting into a sitting position – some useful tips

- Sit on the floor if you can but take it slowly until you are supple enough. Doing yoga will help your body get ready for sitting meditation.

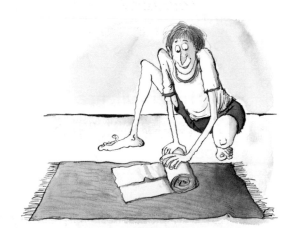

- Always put a folded blanket on the floor to protect your knees and feet.

- You could roll up a blanket to a depth of about 10 cms (4 inches) to sit on.

- Find a sitting position that keeps the back, neck and head in a straight line.

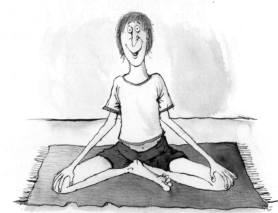

- Try to let go of tension.

- Try to get a solid body position using the two knees and the buttocks

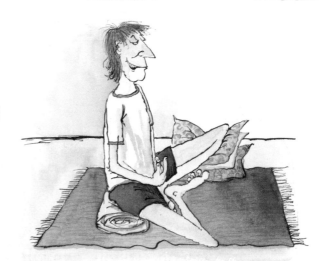

- If the knees do not reach the floor, let them rest on a cushion or pad.

- When the legs are in place, lean forwards once, and with the hands pull the fat of the buttocks out and back.

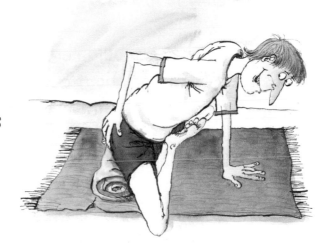

- Then straighten up.

Sitting can be helped by a small round cushion called a **zafu**. You may be able to make a zafu yourself.

Some people like to use a **meditation bench**, which you may also be able to make.

For instructions on making a zafu or meditation bench turn to **pages 46-49** at the end of this section.

While you are sitting ....

- Try to sit tall, as if you want to touch the ceiling with the top of your head. Keep your chin tucked in slightly. This really helps.

- All senses should remain open. Keep your eyes resting on a spot on the floor about a metre from your nose. When you meditate well the eyes will sometimes go out of focus.

- Keep your mouth closed and your jaw relaxed.

- Keep your hands open and place the back of your left hand in the palm of your right.

- The middle knuckles should touch and your thumbs meet.

- Pull your thumbs towards the body to form an oval. This hand position is called a mudra. Energy can flow round this circle and is sealed in by the contact between the hands.

- You may find that you lean a bit when you meditate. Try not to. Gently straighten up if you notice it.

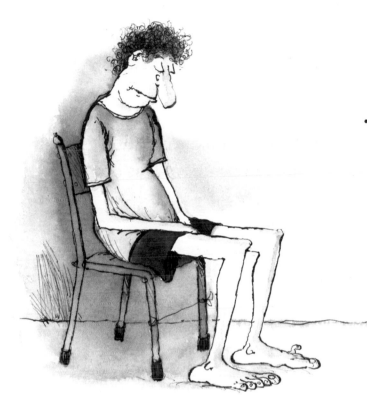

- Try not to slouch!
  It causes distractions.

- Above all let go of your tension!

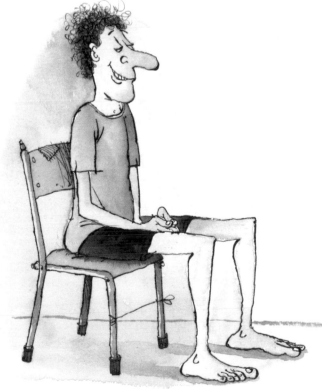

29

'Half Lotus' is a good position to start with

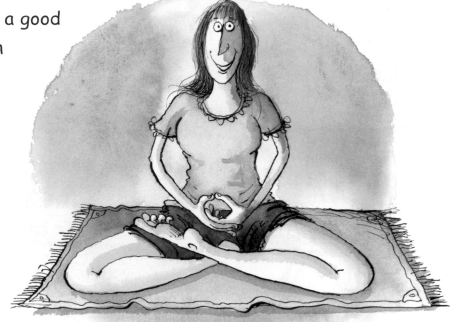

How to get into Half Lotus :-

1. Put your legs straight out in front

2. Bend the right knee and tuck the right foot in close to your body

3. Take the left foot in your right hand

4. Push the left knee to the floor

5. Place the left foot on the right thigh

6. Check you are sitting straight on the zafu

You can also start on the other side by bending the left knee .

'Full Lotus' may be difficult at first, but Yogis often sit in this position. They say that all activity starts on the right side of the body. If you want to silence the body you have to start by 'pinning down' the right side.

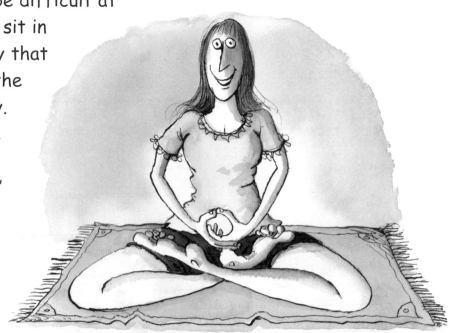

How to get into Full Lotus :-

1. Place the zafu at the back of a folded blanket.

2. Sit on the front half of the zafu with your legs straight out in front.

3. Bend the left knee and tuck the left foot under the right thigh.

4. Bend your right knee. Take the right foot in hand, push the right knee to the floor and place the right foot on the thigh of the left leg.

5. Now bring up the left foot and place it on the right thigh.

Other possible ways to sit are:-

Burmese – with both legs lying bent and parallel on the mat

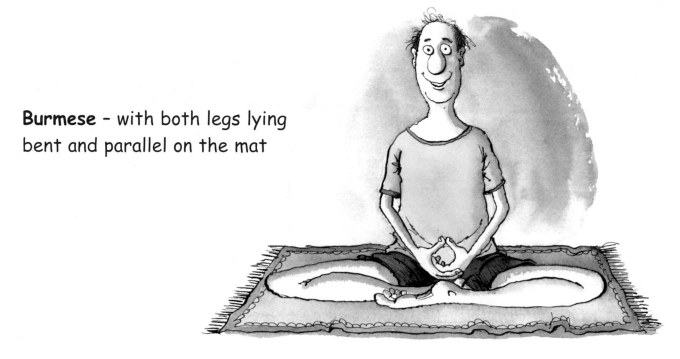

A meditation bench – tuck a rectangular bench under the thighs and buttocks

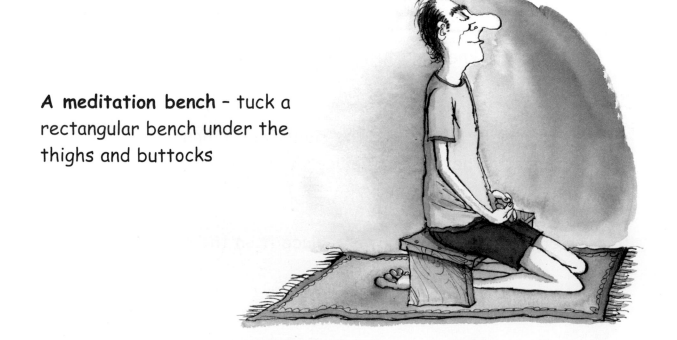

Seiza – sit in a kneeling position on 2 zafus or thicker rolled up blankets

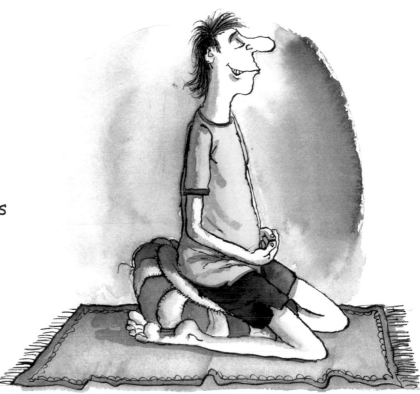

Chair – use the chair as if it were a stool and don't lean on its back

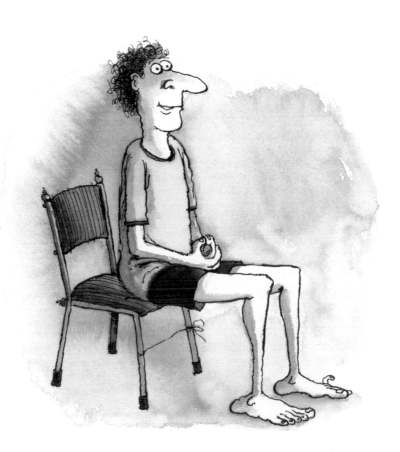

How to silence the mind with breath counting

When the mind concentrates on one-point – the counting of the breath - it will slowly stop running away with itself like a wild horse. This will not happen instantly. Bo Lozoff says in **We're All Doing Time** (page 30)

"We may have to sit through intense periods of terror, lust, perversion, fantasy, grief, guilt, greed, pride, loneliness....... whatever furniture happens to be stored away in here......taking up our peace"

When we become aware of these feelings and thoughts, we just allow them to be and gently return our full focus onto counting the breath.

We learn not to get sucked into the garbage of these distractions. We can always return to the breath.

It can get frustrating at times but that's just one more distraction!

With time our resistance melts. So do our demons!

Counting the breath

- Breathe naturally and watch the breath.

- Never try to breathe differently.

- Count each in-breath and each out-breath up to 10. The first in-breath is 1, the first out-breath is 2, the second in-breath is 3, the second out-breath is 4 and so on.

- Once you have reached 10 go back to 1. Slowly you become aware that you and your breath are one.

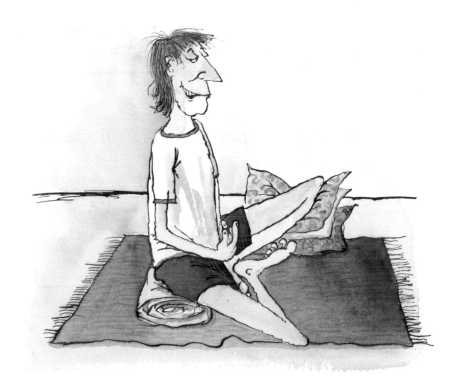

Try an 8 week programme of meditation like this –

Weeks 1 and 2	Count each in-breath and each out-breath as above.
Weeks 3 and 4	Just count the in-breaths and breathe out naturally.
Weeks 5 and 6	Breathe in naturally and count the out-breaths up to 10.
Weeks 7 and 8	Don't count. Sink into silence with each in-breath and out-breath. This is difficult but give it a try.

Try to spend 5 or 10 minutes each time you meditate

From now on ...

When you notice the effects of this programme you may want to sit longer. Slowly extend your meditation to 25 minutes. Early morning is best when the mind is clearer. Sit then, and again in the evening. You will feel the benefit quite soon.

Focus on the breath the way you did for weeks 5 and 6, when you breathed in naturally and counted the out-breaths.

You may also be able to spend short periods with your mind on the breath without counting. This is very peace giving.

After a while if something in the day crops up and stops you from meditating, you will miss your sitting.

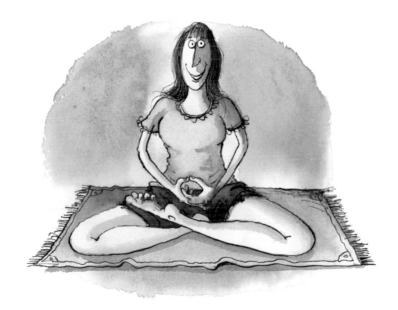

Follow sitting with walking meditation called Kinhin

- Stand up

- Make a fist in the right hand and cover it with the left palm and fingers.

- Rest the eyes on the floor about 1 metre in front.

- Walk slowly letting the leg muscles and tendons flex gently and return the blood flow to normal. This takes about 5 minutes.

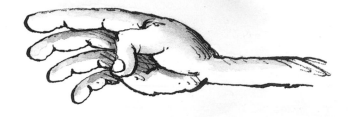
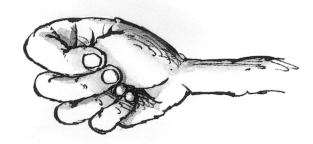

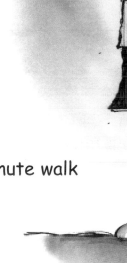

We aim for a 1 hour meditation session!

This is a lot for a beginner.

This is how it goes – 25 minute sit, 5 minute walk
- 25 minute sit, 5 minute walk

Do what you can in your own time.

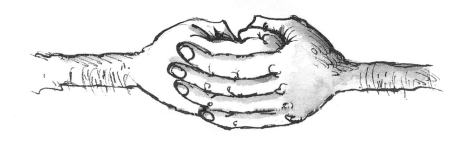

Difficulties you may find in meditating

Fear - people don't often lower their eyes in prison so you may feel afraid at first. But you can create a safe space for yourself. Meditation will become a time when you can leave any fear behind.

Dizziness - Most often this is caused by breathing wrongly. Spend time getting a solid body position so you **'sit like a mountain'**, then breathe <u>naturally</u> - not too deeply, not too slowly.

A Buzz - a buzz alters your consciousness. It is not a good idea to seek a buzz in the hope of enjoyment. During meditation, when anything other than breath awareness enters the mind, gently bring your mind back to your natural breath.

Drugs also alter your consciousness. In the past drugs have been used for spiritual and medicinal purposes but always with guidance. We are sometimes asked if we think drugs can help in meditation. The answer is **NO**. Drugs cut down the power of concentration.

Meditation may help kick drug habits. Getting proper treatment for drug problems and supporting this with meditation would be a sensible thing to do.

Inner noise - At some point breath counting may become too noisy for you. Then you are ready to sit BE-ING the breath. If you have come this far then you will understand what this means and be able to do it. Well done. You are on the way to finding out who you are.

The effects of meditation

The masters of old say that if we meditate regularly and well:

- Our energies that have been all over the place, come together

- We start to gain some control over our super-active minds.

- Tension is released.

- Nerves become relaxed.

- Our health begins to improve.

- We become more aware of our emotions.

- Our will gets stronger.

- We begin to feel an inner balance.

- Gradually our hang-ups melt away.

- Compassion, serenity, selflessness and concern for others come to us more easily.

The first thing we usually notice after regular practice is that we feel refreshed after sitting. Later this seems to deepen into a change of attitude.

We start to see the world as a brighter place. We begin to feel good about ourselves and our lives.

As we feel better we see other people and things that happen day to day as being part of something special and sacred.

Finally we come to a flash of knowing who we really are.

This is a moment of great joy. No matter what your past was, what you have done and what you haven't done.... you are ecstatic and humbled about WHO you really are.

In the East this is called the time when you '**see your own Nature**'. Everyone who sits in silent meditation is on that Path. Sooner or later they will come to the experience if they keep trying.

Remember NOW you have the time!

Use it!

Suggested prayers before and after sitting

Before sitting (from Psalm 40)

I don't want your sacrifices, I want your love. I don't want your offerings, I want you to know me.

Be still and know that I am God. Let us press on to knowing, and God will respond to us as surely as the coming of dawn or the rain of early spring.

After sitting (St. Francis of Assisi)

Make me an instrument of peace.
Where there is hatred, let me sow love.
Where there is injury, pardon.
Where there is doubt, faith.
Where there is despair, hope.
Where there is darkness, light.
Where there is sadness, joy.

Let me not so much seek to be consoled as to console,
Not so much to be understood, as to understand,
Not so much to be loved, as to love.
For it is in giving that we receive,
It is in forgiving that we are pardoned,
And it is in dying that we are born to eternal life.

When all of us at the Trust sit each morning in meditation, we hold all of you in our hearts and remember you in our prayers.

Please believe that every time you practice yoga or meditation, **we are with you**.

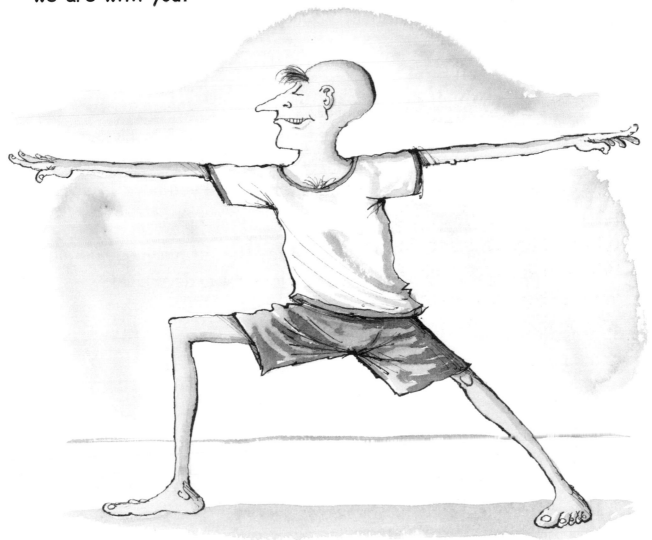

How to make a zafu and meditation bench

How to make a zafu

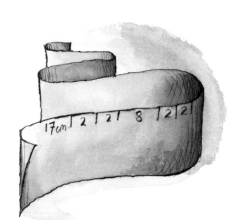

1. Take a length of cloth about 1.5 meters long and 16cms wide.

2. Pleat the length of cloth.

    a) Start 17cms from the left end and make 3 marks each 2cms apart. 8cms after this set make another 3 marks 2cms apart and so on every 8cms until you have 14 sets of pleat markings.

    b) Fold the 3rd marking in to meet the 1st marking and pin. Pin all pleats always folding cloth towards the left.

3. Take the right end of the pleated cloth and overlap the left end by 8cms. Pin the overlap.

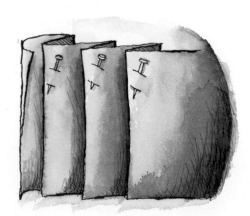

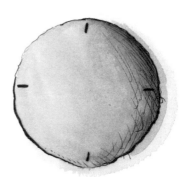
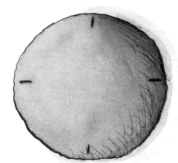

4. Cut two circles of cloth with
    a diameter of 30.5cms.

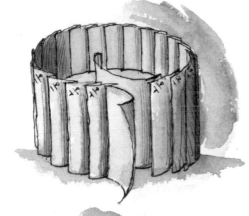

5. Pin in one circle to the pleated strip
    at the top and one at the bottom.

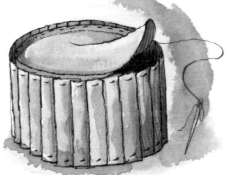

6. Ease the pleats into the circle and
    stitch.

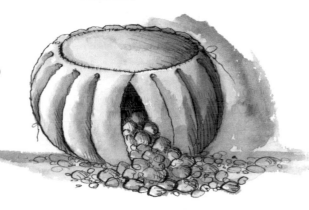

7. Turn inside out and stuff with a
    mixture of foam chips and kapok to
    the right height for you.

47

How to make a meditation bench

You need a plank about 2cm thick, 15cm wide, 82cm long

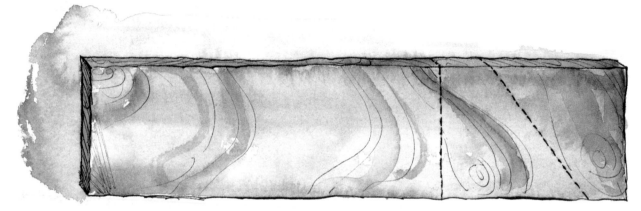

Saw it into 3 pieces

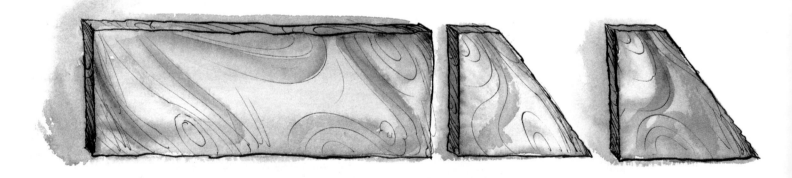

You can put it together with metal 90 brackets OR wooden pegs and glue OR with screws.

It isn't strong enough if you just use nails.

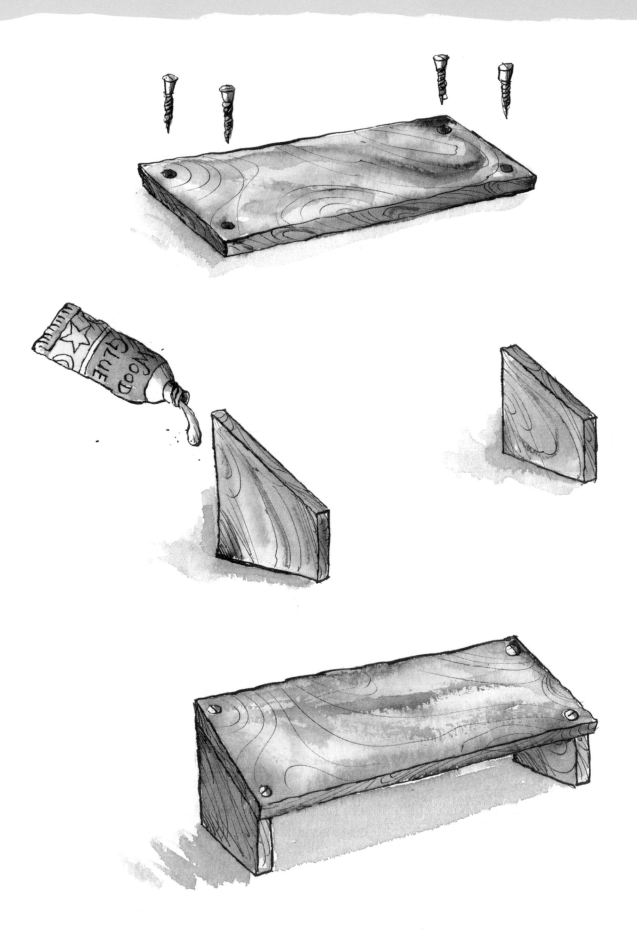

List of yoga poses - Asanas

Corpse pose   page 52

Wind-releasing pose   page 54

The Bridge   page 56

Floor Twist   page 58

Cobbler's pose   page 60

Frog pose   page 62

Cat pose   page 64

Mountain pose   page 66

Moving Mountain pose   page 67

Triangle pose   page 68

Warrior pose   page 70

Stretched Flank pose   page 72

Tree pose   page 74

Shoulder-stands   page 76

Fish pose   page 82

Sun Salutation   page 84

Yoga poses – Asanas

Health and Safety

- **Before you start your yoga, you need to warm-up.** One way to do this is to 'run-on-the-spot' but without lifting your feet off the floor. Bend the right knee and take the heel of the right foot off the ground at the same time. Place heel back on the floor and lift left heel up. Pick up speed as you move from right to left, pumping your arms as you go.

- **Do check that it is safe for you to do a pose.** Look in the 'WATCH IT!' section under each pose to make sure it is OK for you.

- **When you are told to repeat a pose on the other side it is important to do this.** It balances the body. If you don't do this you become lop-sided and can injure yourself.

- **It is important to come out of a pose safely.** If you focus on your breath this is easy. This is how:-

'breathe in and **move out of the pose** on the **out-breath**'.

CORPSE POSE

HOW TO DO IT:

1. Lie flat on your back with your arms on the floor. Your hands are a foot away from your hips, palms facing up. Check your body and head are in a straight line. Tuck your chin in gently. Let your feet fall apart either side of an imaginary central line. Relax everything – your feet, your legs, your trunk, your arms and hands, your neck and head. Close your eyes gently and breathe easily. Relax and let go.

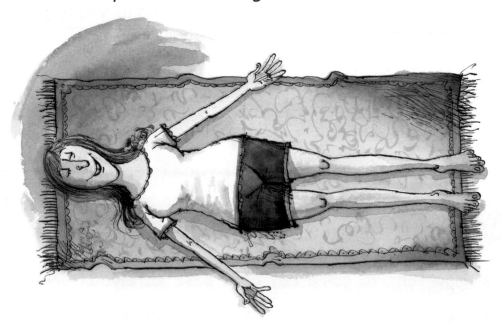

2. Try not to move at all even if you get a bit uncomfortable.

3. Breathe naturally. Let the mind receive the breath as it comes in and out. It may help to count each out-breath until you reach 10. Then you can start again at '1'. Gradually you, your body, mind, spirit and breath become one. Then the breathing becomes fine and you can just BE.

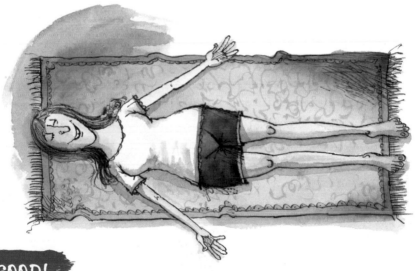

THIS IS GOOD!

• helps relax you before and after yoga practice
• helps calm and restore body and mind
• helps reduce stress and high blood pressure
• helps develop body awareness
• helps improve sleep

Time: 3-5 minutes minimum

WIND-RELEASING POSE

HOW TO DO IT:

1. Lie flat on your back resting your head on the floor.

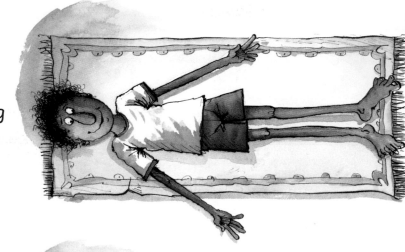

2. Bend your right leg up to your chest and interlock your fingers over the knee, bringing your right thigh in close towards your chest.

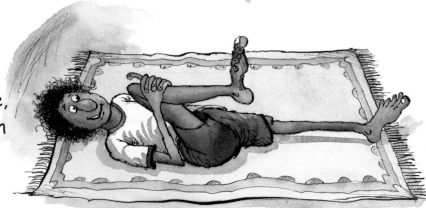

3. Breathe in and breathe out. In the pause, while you are empty of breath, lift your head and try to touch your knee with your nose.

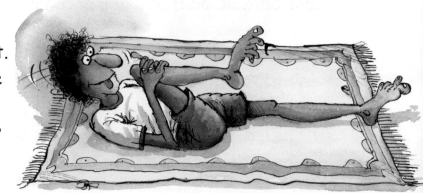

4. Breathe in and rest your head
    back down on the floor.
    Do this slowly 5-10 times.

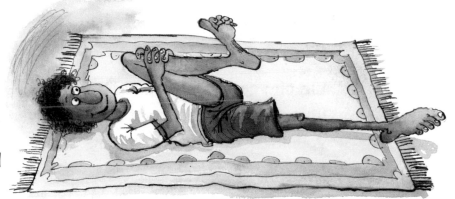

5. Switch your legs round
    and repeat.

6. Then bring both your knees onto
    your chest and wrap your arms
    around your knees. Keep your
    head on the floor as you rest.

When holding 2 legs keep your knees apart if it is more
comfortable or if you are pregnant.

THIS IS GOOD!

- helps relieve wind and
  constipation
- helps relieve back-ache

WATCH IT!

- don't do this if you have
  sciatica or a slipped disc

THE BRIDGE POSE

HOW TO DO IT:

1. Lie on your back, your knees bent up and your feet apart on the floor, your heels near to buttocks. Arms rest on the floor by your sides.

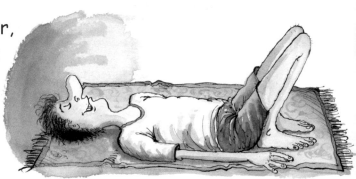

2. Breathe in. Slowly breathe out pressing the back of your waist into the floor, tilting your pelvis and pubic bone up. Squeeze the buttock muscles. Pause.

3. Breathe in and lift your buttocks and back high off the floor, taking your arms up and back behind you to lie alongside your ears. Pause.

4. Breathe out. As you do so bring back your arms to the ground and lower your spine, bone by bone down onto the floor. Try to get your waist on the floor before you lengthen out your lower back.

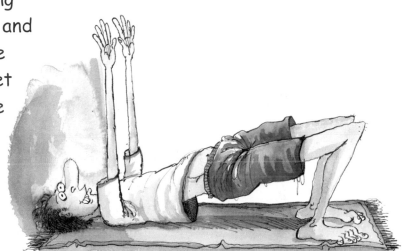

5. Breathe in and relax completely.

6. Repeat these 4 movements 6 times.

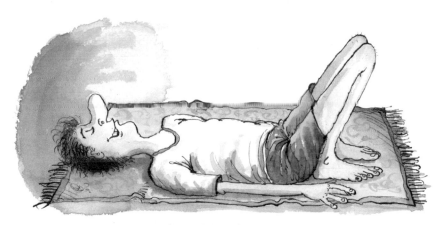

THIS IS GOOD!

- helps relieve back-ache
- helps improve breathing
- helps wake up whole body

WATCH IT!

- don't do this if you have an injured back
- don't do this if you have stomach ulcers

57

FLOOR TWISTS

HOW TO DO IT:

1. Lie on your back with your knees on your chest.

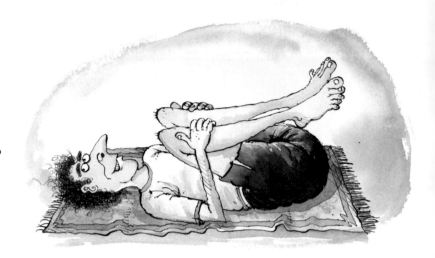

2. Breathe in slowly then as you breathe out roll over onto your right side. Your arms should be straight out in front of you, palms together. Relax completely as though you were in bed at night.

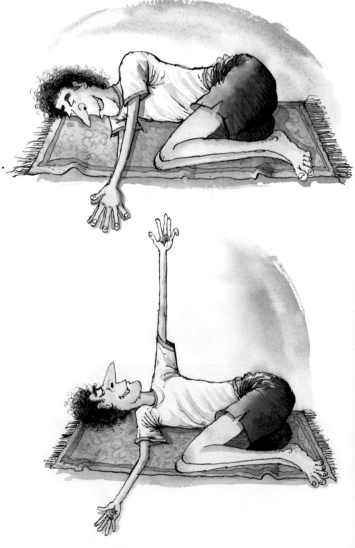

3. On an in-breath, extend your left arm up in the air. Turning your head and looking at your hand at all times, bring the arm over to the floor, level with the shoulder on your left side.

4. Your ribs move to the left and your hips and knees continue to point towards the right.

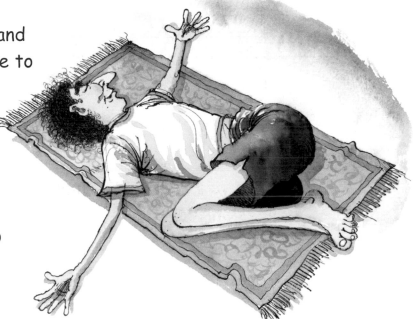

5. Sink your left shoulder into the floor. Relax.

6. Breathe slowly up to 10 breaths.

7. Repeat on the other side.

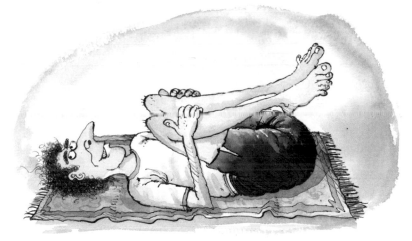

THIS IS GOOD!

- helps back-ache
- helps indigestion
- helps to realign back-bones

COBBLER'S POSE

HOW TO DO IT:

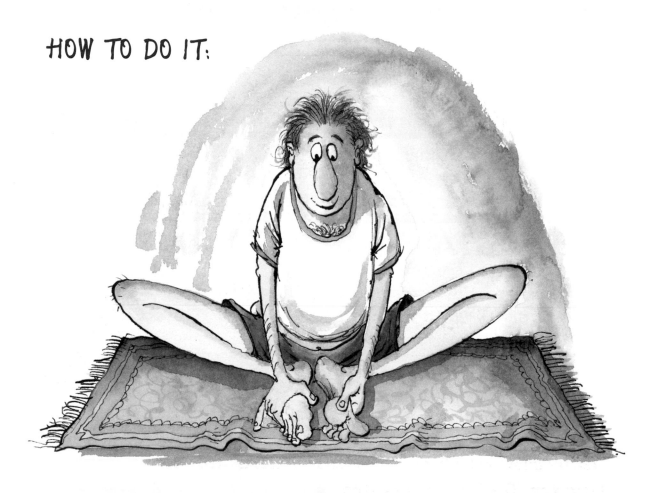

1. Sit upright and bring the soles of your feet together and your heels as close to your groin as you can.

2. Interlock your fingers and clasp your hands around your toes.

3. Use your feet for leverage, lift your chest forward and straighten your spine.

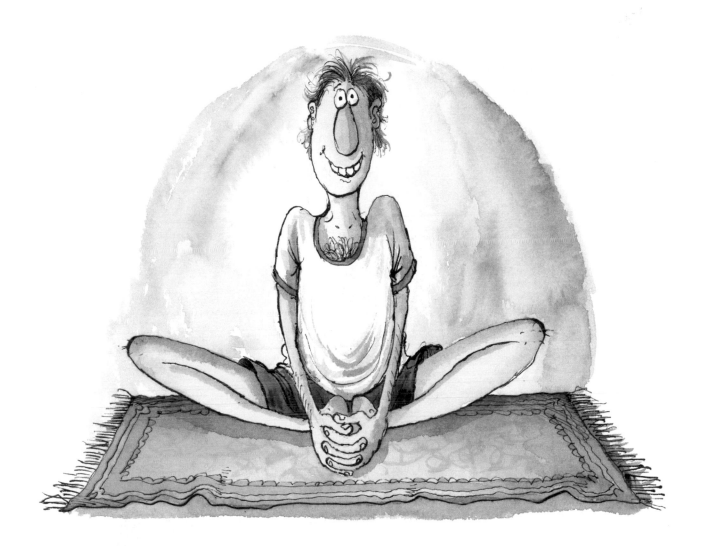

4. Gently allow your knees to release towards the floor.
   Hold for 10 – 20 easy breaths.

THIS IS GOOD!

- helps loosen groin and hip muscles
- helps open rib-cage

WATCH IT!

- don't do this if you have sciatica or low back problems

61

FROG POSE

HOW TO DO IT:

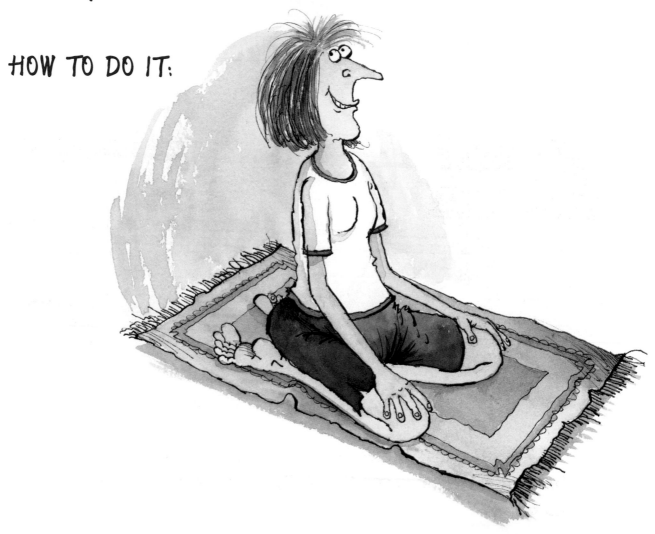

1. Kneel upright with your knees apart as far as is comfortable. Keep your feet flat on the floor. Keep your buttocks on your heels.

2. Lean forward until your hands touch the floor. Continue to bend forwards until your arms are stretched along the floor. Let your chest sink down until your forehead rests on the floor.

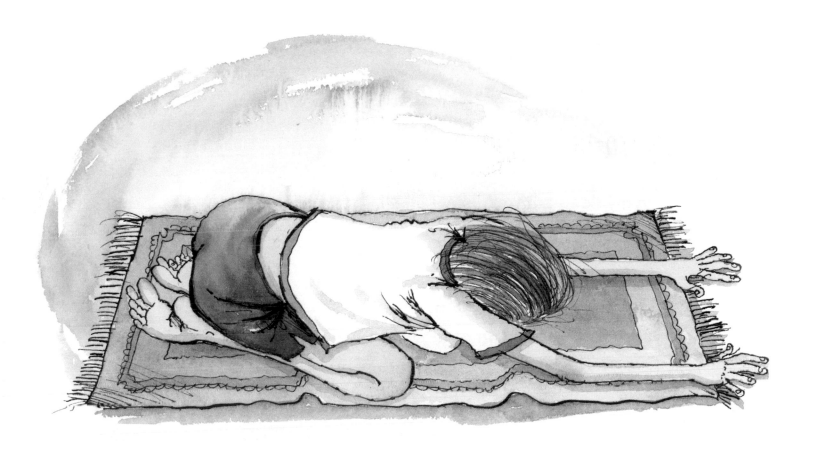

3. Your ribs and chest are free to breathe easily.

4. At first your groin may feel tight and you may only want to breathe slowly 3 times. Gradually as you learn to relax you can do more.

THIS IS GOOD!

- helps improve breathing
- helps relax tight groin and back muscles
- helps deep calm

63

CAT POSE

HOW TO DO IT:

1. On a folded blanket, kneel on all fours with your hands shoulder width apart and your knees hip width apart. With your head level in a straight line with your spine, look down at a spot on the floor below your navel. Breathe in.

2. Breathe out, tucking your tail-bone under, arching your back and bringing your chin down to the chest to squeeze out the last of the air. Draw back your belly muscles and feel as though you can pull up everything inside from between the legs. Pause, empty of breath.

64

3. Breathe in, turning your tail-bone up,
   hollowing your back and bringing
   your head in line with your spine.
   If you can, look up. Let your belly
   muscles fall towards the floor.
   Pause full of breath.
   Then begin again.

4. Repeat the arching movements as you breathe in and out.

THIS IS GOOD!

- helps bring flexibility to spine, neck, and shoulders
- helps tone the nervous system
- helps digestion
- helps us find a sense of calm

MOUNTAIN POSE

HOW TO DO IT:

1. Stand with your feet together. Feel the floor beneath your feet and adjust your weight evenly. Lift the front of your chest, and relax your shoulders. Feel an invisible string pulling you up from the top of your head. Look at the floor in front of you. Breathe deeply. Continue for 10-20 breaths.

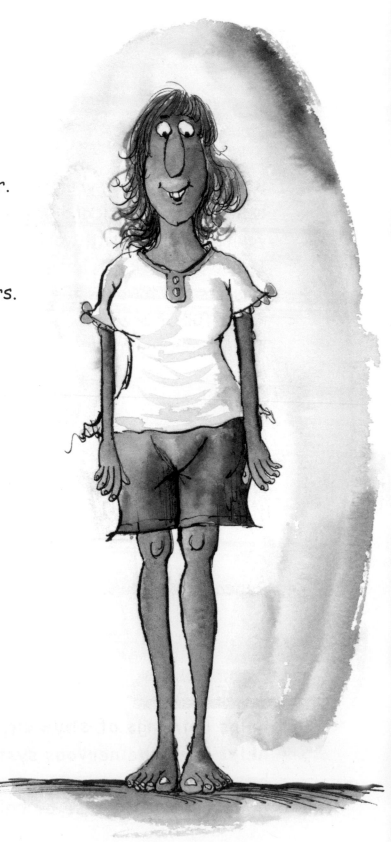

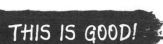

THIS IS GOOD!

- helps lift the spirits
- helps with good posture

MOVING MOUNTAIN

HOW TO DO IT:

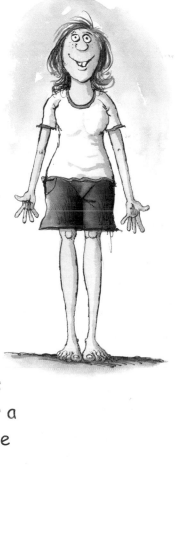

1. Stand with your arms by your sides, palms facing forward.

2. As you breathe in, try to allow the breath to lift your arms above your head until the palms meet. Remain full of breath for a couple of seconds. When you are ready, allow the out-breath to lower your arms to your sides.

3. Repeat 5-10 times.

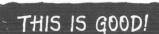
THIS IS GOOD!

- helps rid lungs of stale air and replace with fresh
- helps wake up body

TRIANGLE POSE

HOW TO DO IT:

1. This pose looks simple but feels hard. Stand with your legs leg-length apart. Turn your left toes in, and your right toes out. Your hips face forward. Your spine is straight. Relax.

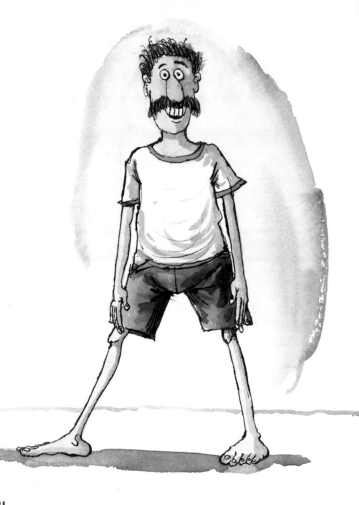

2. Raise your arms to shoulder-height. Relax your shoulders even though your arms are raised! Breathe in and out easily as you stretch from finger-tip to finger-tip.

3. Breathe in, and breathing out stretch over to the right. Continue breathing.

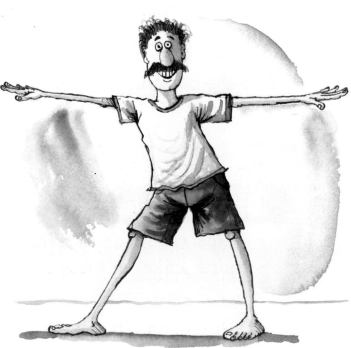

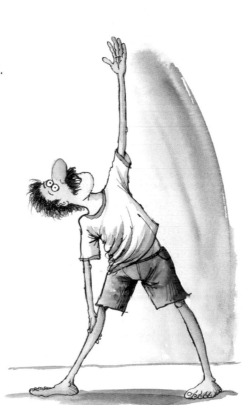

4. Lower your right arm and right side until your right hand rests on your right leg somewhere below the knee (or lower if you can).

5. Lift your left arm until it points up in a straight line with your right arm. If you can, look up to the raised hand, where the palm faces forward. Try to keep your left hip back.

6. Breathe calmly for 3-5 breaths.

7. Take care to use the breath to come out of this pose – breathe in and move out of the pose on the out-breath.

8. Repeat on the other side.

THIS IS GOOD!

- helps lift spirits
- helps improve digestion
- helps release stiffness in feet, ankles and hips
- helps open rib-cage

WATCH IT!

- don't do this if you have a painful lower back

WARRIOR POSE

HOW TO DO IT:

1. Stand with your feet really wide apart.

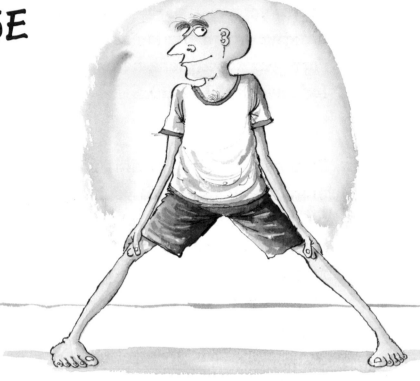

2. Turn your left toes in and your right toes out. Keep your left leg straight and bend your right knee until it ends up directly above your right ankle. Try to sink your right thigh down. Keep the outside edge of the left foot grounded. Try to keep your spine straight. With your legs strong – relax!

3. Raise your arms to shoulder level. Relax your shoulders. Breathe easily. Stretch from fingertip to fingertip. Turn your head to look along your right arm. Breathe deeply and calmly for 3-5 breaths.

4. To come out of this pose, lower the arms, breathe in and move out of the pose on the out-breath. Heel-toe or jump legs together if you wish.

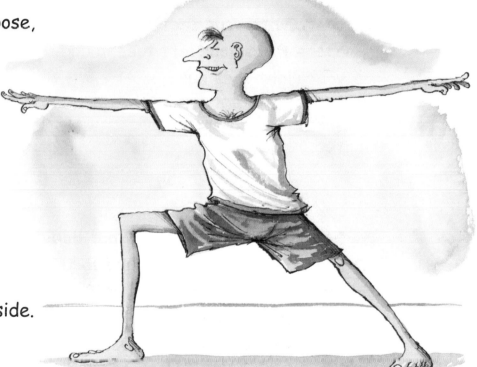

5. Repeat on the other side.

THIS IS GOOD!

- helps open and loosen shoulder joints
- helps increase lung capacity and circulation
- helps strengthen legs and open hips
- helps people keep their feet on the ground!

WATCH IT!

- don't do this if you have arthritic hips

71

STRETCHED FLANK POSE

HOW TO DO IT:

1. Stand with your feet really wide apart. Point your left toes in and your right toes out.

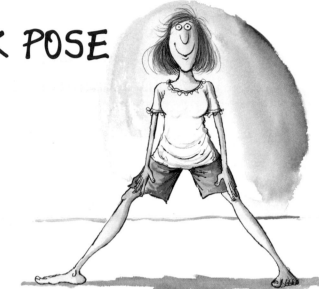

2. Stretch the left side of your body by lowering your right hand to the floor to the big-toe side of your right foot, using your right arm to keep the right knee back.

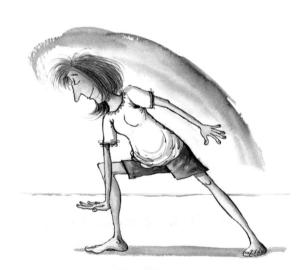

3. Turn your upper body and head to look at the ceiling so that your rib-cage faces up.

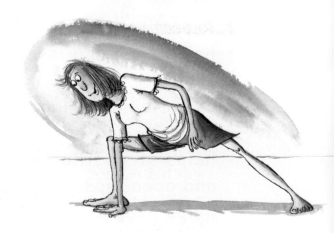

4. Lift your left arm up and stretch it to the right until it is over your left ear. Try to look in front of your upper arm at the ceiling. Breathe easily and relax.

5. Relax your face. Hold for 3 – 5 breaths.

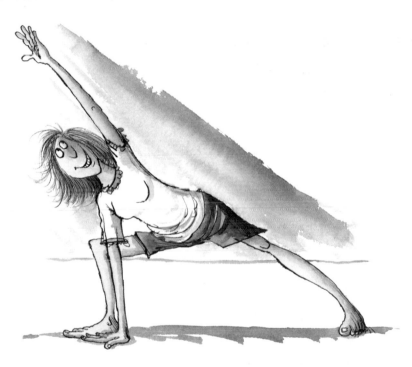

6. Take care getting out of this pose. First lower your arm then breathe in and move out of the pose on the out-breath.

7. Repeat on the other side.

THIS IS GOOD!

- helps internal organs work better
- helps trim and lengthen the waist

WATCH IT!

- don't do this if you have arthritic hips

TREE POSE

HOW TO DO IT:

1. Stand with your chin level or slightly down. Focus on and keep looking at a spot on the floor – this will help you to balance. Shift your weight onto your left leg as you soften your right knee.

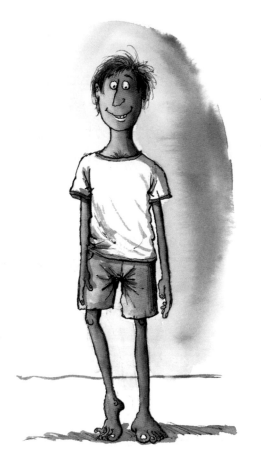

2. Bend your right knee. Place your right foot against your left thigh, high up in the groin.

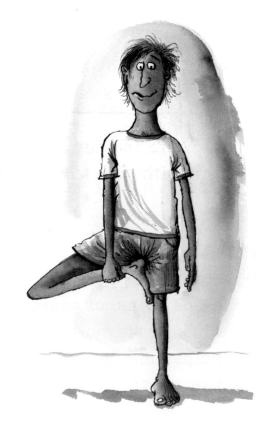

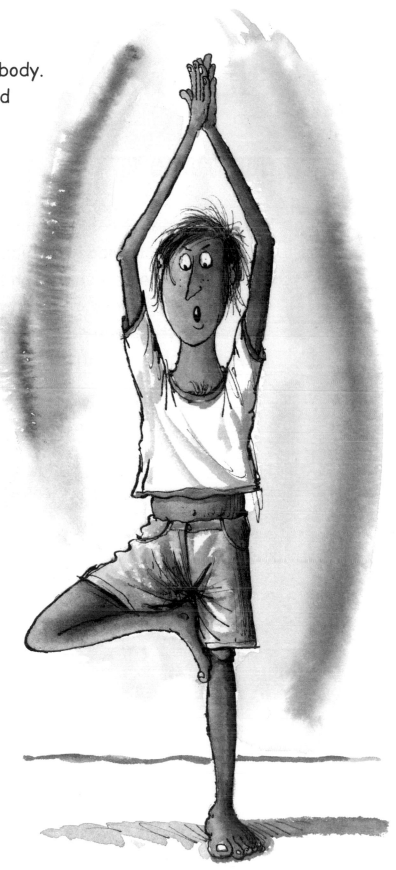

3. Breathe easily and settle the body. Raise your arms over your head until the palms of your hands come together.

4. Don't worry if you wobble. Hold for 5 – 10 easy breaths.

5. Repeat on the other leg.

Easier options:

- place your right foot on your left foot
- place the arch of your right foot on the inside knee of your left leg
- hang onto the wall
- try it with bare legs and feet

THIS IS GOOD!

- helps concentration
- helps inner balance

A. FULL SHOULDER-STAND

HOW TO DO IT:

1. Fold a blanket to give a height of 2 or 3 inches (4cm). Lie on your back on the blanket with your arms by your sides and your shoulders in line with the edge of the blanket. The back of your head and neck rest on the floor, free of the blanket. **The blanket is important to prevent your neck from injury.**

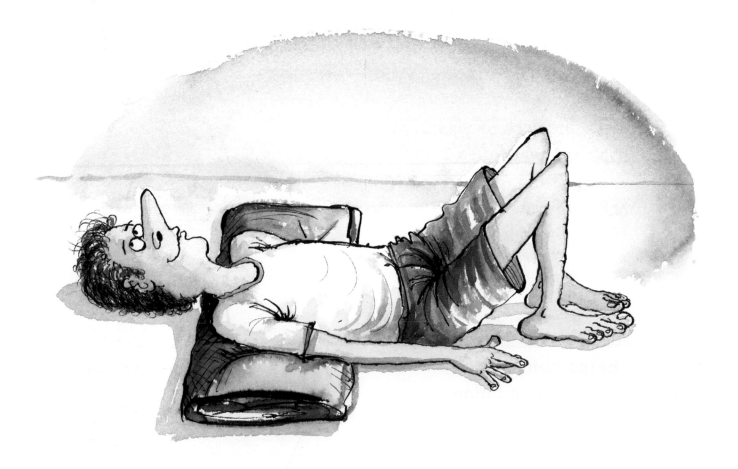

2. Breathe in. Breathing out, swing your knees over your chest.

3. Breathe in. Breathing out, swing your knees over your forehead. Lift your hips from the floor and support the top of your buttocks with your hands. Breathe easily.

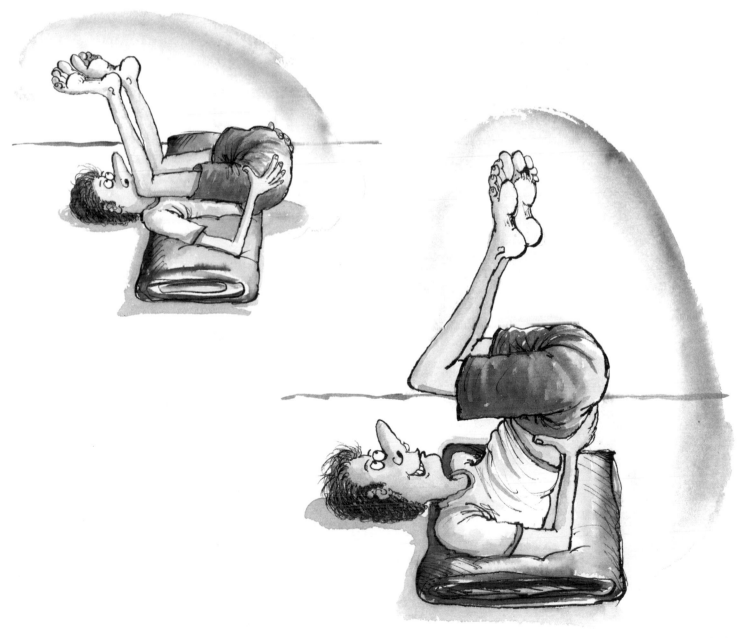

A. FULL SHOULDER-STAND continued ...

4. Straighten and extend your legs upwards.

5. Walk your hands down your back towards your shoulder blades. Lift your chest towards your chin. Breathe easily. Relax any muscles not in use. Hold pose for 10 breaths. Later on, you can hold it for 3-5 minutes.

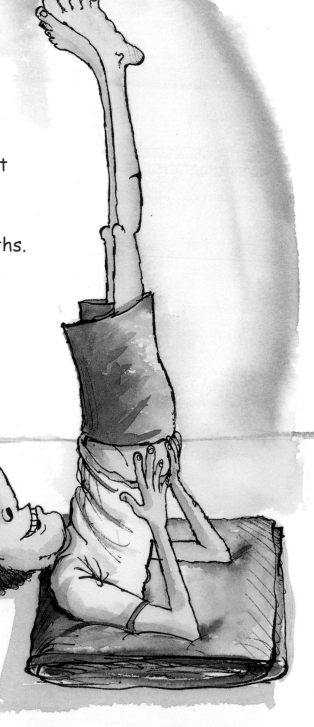

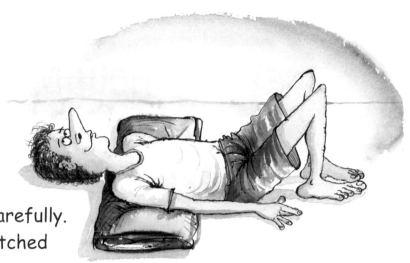

6. To release, lower yourself carefully. Rest for a few breaths stretched along the floor before sitting up.

THIS IS GOOD!

- helps people sleep better
- helps relieve anxiety
- helps reduce headaches
- helps heal and relax the body and mind
- helps prevent colds and flu

WATCH IT!

- don't do this if you have high blood pressure or heart condition
- don't do this if you have neck or back injury
- don't do this if you have detached retina or glaucoma
- don't do this if you have hiatus hernia
- don't do this if you have blood-thinning drugs (check with your doctor)
- don't do this if you have a period
- don't do this if you have breathlessness from strong physical exercise

B. EASY SHOULDER-STAND

HOW TO DO IT:

1. Place the edge of a folded blanket against a wall. Lie down on your back with your buttocks and legs up against the wall and your shoulders in line with the edge of the blanket. The back of your head and neck rest on the floor.

2. Bend your knees and place your feet flat on a wall. Using your feet to steady you, lift your hips off the floor and support your back with your hands. Encourage your chest towards your chin. As an easier pose you can stay like this and breathe.

3. If you want to, walk your feet up a wall until your legs are straight and then walk your hands further down your back towards your shoulder blades, lifting the chest. As an easier pose you can stay like this and breathe.

4. To try the full pose, remove your feet from the wall and extend your legs overhead.

1.

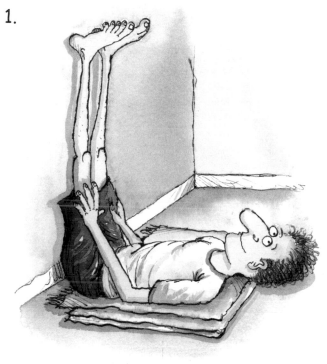

2.

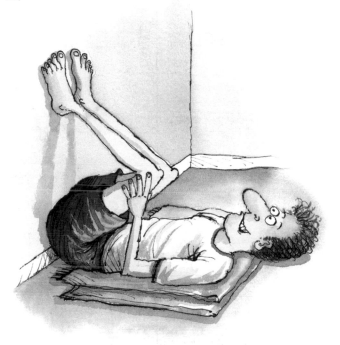

3.

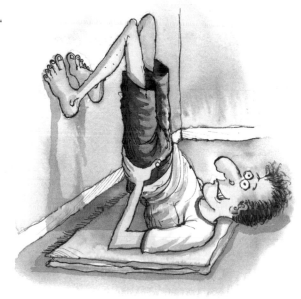

4.

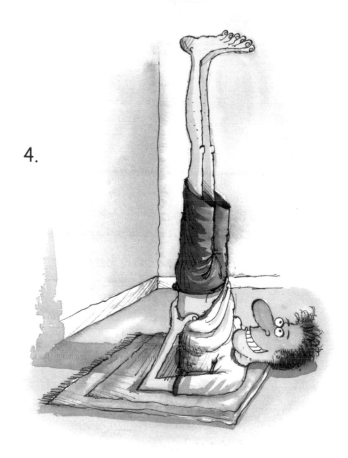

FISH POSE

HOW TO DO IT:

1. Lie on your back on the floor. Stretch your legs out straight and tuck your elbows in close to your body.

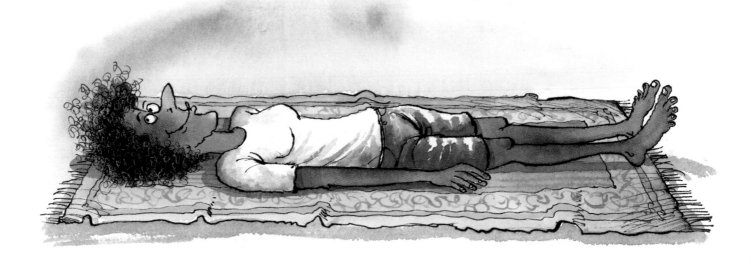

2. Breathe in and keeping your buttocks and head on the floor, push your elbows into the ground and arch your chest upwards.

3. Raise your chin and try to look back at the wall behind you, sliding onto the **top** of your head. Support yourself with your elbows and forearms.

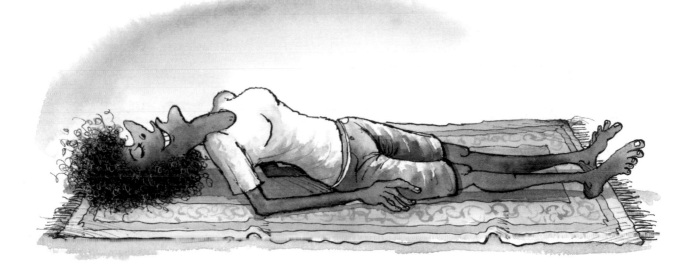

4. Breathe easily. Hold for 3-5 breaths.

THIS IS GOOD!

- helps improve breathing problems
- helps release stiff middle and upper back muscles

WATCH IT!

- don't do this if you have a neck injury

83

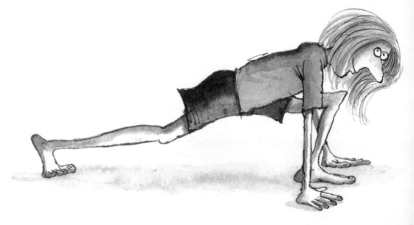

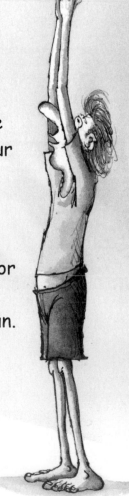

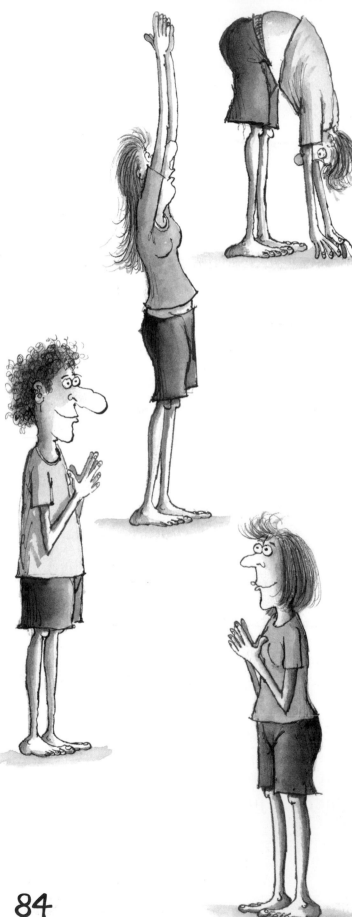

SUN SALUTATION

The beautiful Sun Salutation wakes up the whole body so it is good to do this in the morning.

The 12 flowing movements are linked with the breath – a reminder of our unity with the whole of creation.

Face the sun in your cell if you can - but you can work with the sun's energy whichever way your room faces.

The bowing and arching movements show our reverence and gratitude for our own inner light and for the light of the sun.

84

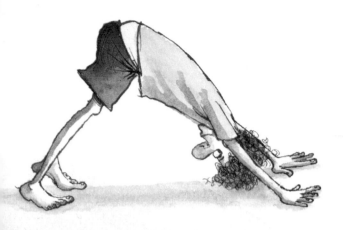

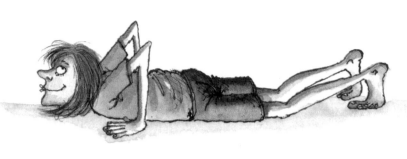

THIS IS GOOD!

- helps loosen and energise the body

WATCH IT!

- don't do this if you have a back injury
- don't do this if you have not warmed up first. If you have not warmed up, take it gently.

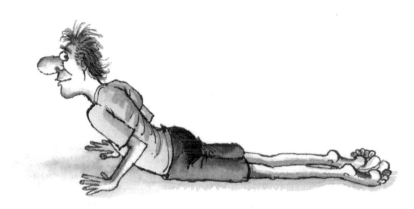

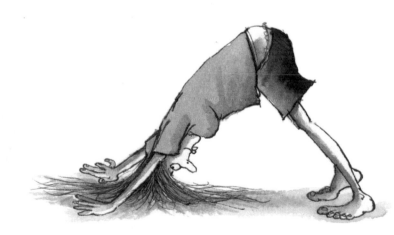

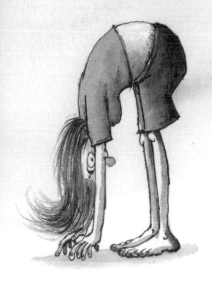

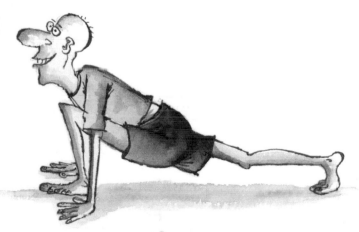

85

SUN SALUTATION

HOW TO DO IT:

Pose 1: Mountain Pose

Stand with your feet together and with your hands in prayer position. Breathe in and breathe out.

Pose 2: Upwards Stretch

Breathing in, raise your arms and look up. Breathing out, open the arms, soften your knees, tuck your tail-bone under and arch your back. Breathe in, straighten and stretch up.

Pose 3: Forward Bend

Breathing out bend forward and bring your hands towards the floor. Release your head from your neck so it moves freely. Bend your knees to get your palms on the floor.

1.

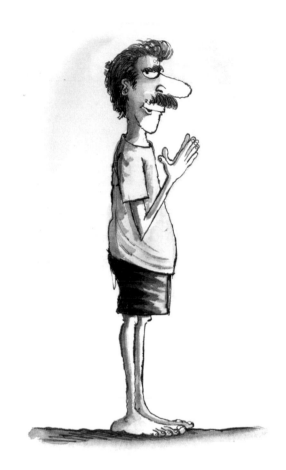

2.

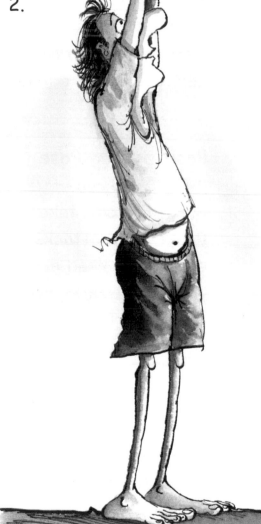

3.

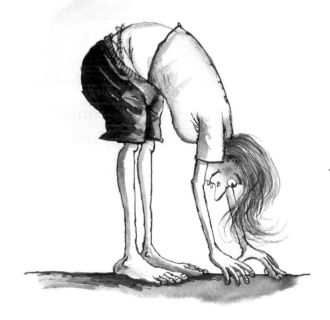

SUN SALUTATION continued ...

Pose 4: Equestrian Pose

Breathing in, take your right leg back behind you. Bend your left knee and bring your hands to the floor either side of your left foot.

Pose 5: Dog Pose

Breathing out, take your left foot back to join your right foot. Raise your buttocks in the air and stretch through your hands and arms. Your head drops freely between your shoulders. Stretch your chest back towards your thighs. Extend the heels down. Keep your legs straight.

Pose 6: Plank Pose

Breathing in, keep your weight on your hands and arms. Lower your buttocks until your body is in a straight line. As in the "press-up" position, lower your body to the floor.

4.

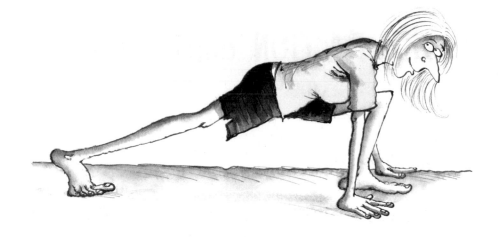

5.

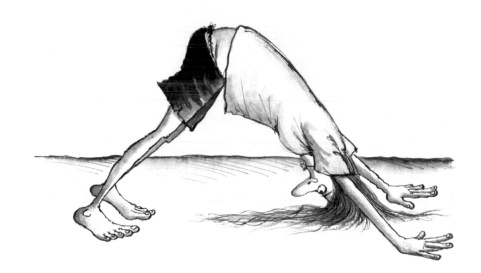

6.

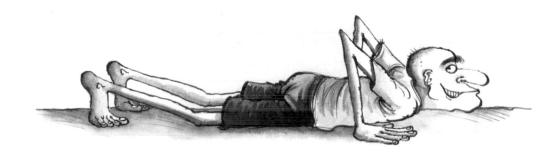

SUN SALUTATION continued ...

Pose 7: Cobra Pose

Keeping the tops of your feet on the floor, breathe out and squeeze your buttock muscles to tuck your tail-bone under. Use the strength of your hands to lift your chest upwards without lifting your hips from the floor. Drop your shoulders away from your ears as you lift your rib-cage. Breathe in.

Pose 8: Dog Pose

Tuck your toes under. Raise your buttocks in the air and stretch through your hands and arms. Your head drops freely between your shoulders. Stretch your chest back towards your thighs. Extend the heels down. Keep your legs straignt (as in Pose 5).

Pose 9: Equestrian Pose

Breathing in swing your right foot forwards between your hands.

7.

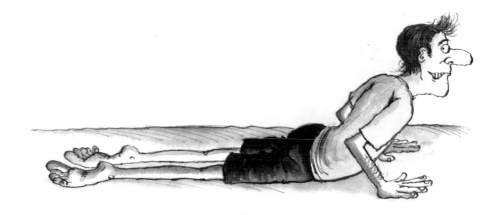

8.

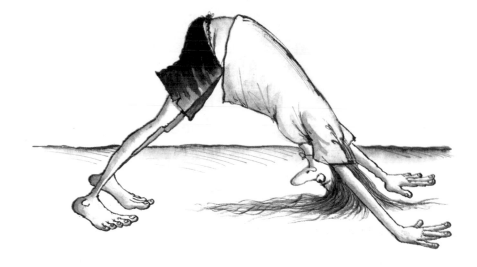

9.

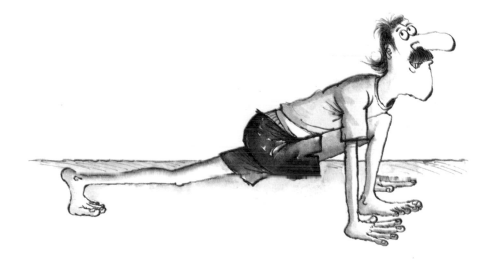

SUN SALUTATION continued ...

Pose 10: Forward Bend

Breathing out swing your left foot forward to join your right foot. Straighten your knees, and hang forward, relaxed like a rag doll.

Pose 11: Upwards Stretch

Breathing in, bend your knees and stretch your arms all the way up. Look up. Breathing out, soften your knees, tuck your tail-bone under and arch your back. Breathe in and straighten (as in Pose 2).

Pose 12: Mountain Pose

Breathing out return your hands to the prayer position.

10.

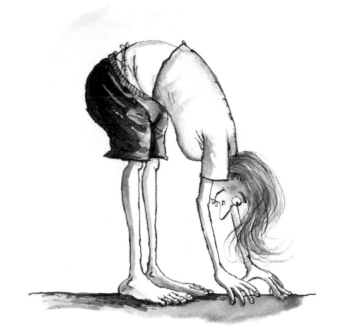

11.

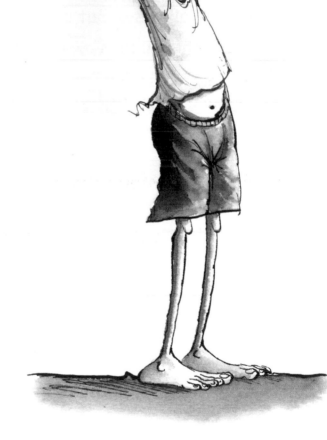

12.

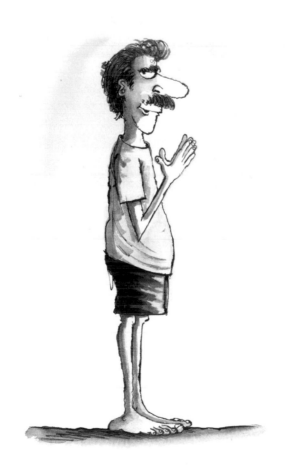

SUN SALUTATION

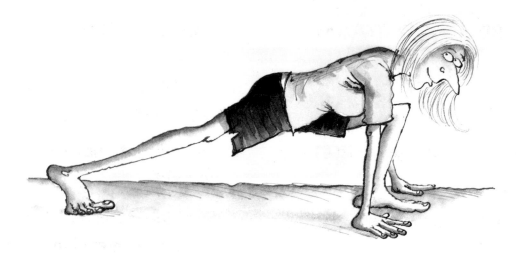

Repeat all poses but start again by taking the **left** leg behind you in Equestrian pose. This makes one complete round.

You can do up to 12 rounds of The Sun Salutation.

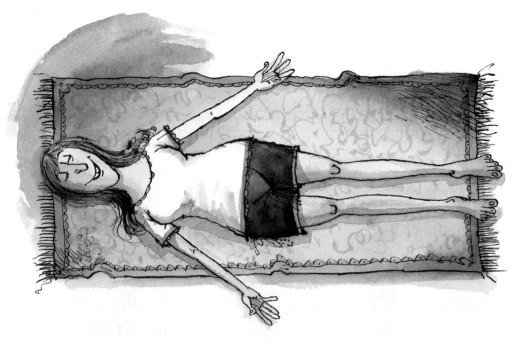

Then.........rest in the Corpse Pose.

94

GLOSSARY

Some words used and their meanings

THE WORD	HOW TO SAY IT	THE MEANING
Asanas	(**Ars** – un – ers)	The Indian word for a Yoga pose
Capacity	(ka- **pas** – it-e)	The amount that can be held
Concentrate	(**kon** – sen - trate)	To think deeply and to focus on something
Contemplation	(**kon** – tem – **play**-shon)	Thinking about something deeply and for a long time
Demons	(**dee** – mons)	Most often bad spiritual influences
Distractions	(dis – **trak** – shons)	Things that take up your mind and get in the way of clear thinking
Ebbing	(**eb** – ing)	Going backwards like the sea
Flowing	(**flo** – ing)	Moving forwards freely and easily like the sea
Frustration	(frus – **tray** – shon)	Feelings of working to no effect

GLOSSARY

Kinhin	(Kin – **hin**)	A way to meditate while walking
Meditation	(med – e – **tay** – shon)	A way of sitting still in silence that can give deep calm.
Phoenix	(**fee**-niks)	We are told that after this bird died in a fire it rose from the ashes as if born again.
Physical	(**fiz** – ik- al)	To do with the body
Pranayama	(pra – na – ya -ma)	How to focus on the breath
Reflection	(re – **flek** – shon)	Careful or long thought
Resistance	(re – **zist** – ance)	The power of something that gets in the way of what we want to do.
Retreat	(re – **treet**)	Time out in a quiet place to think or pray
Revealed	(re – **veeld**)	When something can suddenly be seen clearly
Reverence	(**rev** – er – ence)	Special respect and high regard
Rhythmically	(**rith** – mik - al - ee)	With a regular movement or beat

GLOSSARY

Sacred	(**say** – kred)	Something special and holy which we feel at home with but can't find the words for
Seiza	(**say**-sa)	Kneeling position
Sheltered	(**shel** – terd)	Protected from the wind, weather or from outside problems
Sociable	(**So** – she – a - bl)	Friendly and liking the company of other people
Spiritual	(**spir**- it- yew - al)	Having feelings and thoughts which make us feel connected and fully alive
Smouldering	(**smole** – der – ing)	Burning slowly without a flame
Supple	(**sup** – pl)	Easy to bend
Tension	(**ten** – shon)	Feelings of being pulled tight with anxiety and stress
Upanishads	(oo – **pan** – ish – ads)	Ancient Indian teachings.
Zafu	(**za** – fu)	A round meditation cushion
Zen	(zen)	Silent meditation which in time reveals our true selves

About the contributors to this book

The authors

Sandy Chubb, Director of the Prison Phoenix Trust, has worked as a yoga and meditation teacher for 30 years. She taught young offenders at HMYOI Aylesbury before working for the PPT where she now teaches prisoners all over the UK and Eire. Sandy studies meditation with the Oxford Zen Centre.

Sister Elaine MacInnes directs Freeing the Human Spirit – a charity which establishes meditation and yoga classes in Canadian prisons. She is a Catholic nun and former Prison Phoenix Trust Director. She studied meditation under Zen Buddhist Masters in Japan and became a Zen master herself.

The editor

Susanna Lee studied Forensic and Legal Psychology and has another degree in African and Asian and Religious Studies. She taught literacy and communication skills to young offenders and adults in prisons and to young people in colleges and the community. Susanna has practiced yoga for many years.

The designer

Nicola Kenwood studied a degree in Visual Communication Design at Ravensbourne College. She set up her own design company, Hakoona Matata, where she specialises in designing children's educational books for publishers such as Harper Collins, whose 'Big Cat' series won the BESA Education Award for Primary Books in 2005.

The illustrator

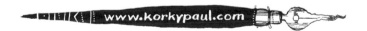

Korky Paul was born in Zimbabwe and studied Fine Art at Durban Art School, South Africa. Later he studied Film Animation in California. Korky has illustrated many well-known children's books including the "Winnie the Witch" series which won the Children's Book Award.

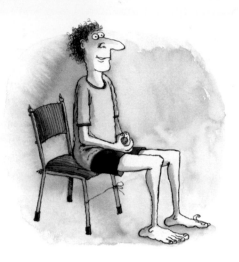

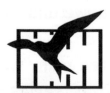

THE PRISON PHOENIX TRUST
PO Box 328 Oxford OX2 7HF

www.prisonphoenixtrust.org.uk